Intermittent Fasting

How to Gain More Muscle, Optimize Fat Loss, and Achieve a Super-Human Focus

I0447760

Table Of Contents

Introduction

I want to thank you and congratulate you for purchasing the book, "Intermittent Fasting: Learning about its benefits for diet, weight loss and overall health".

This book aims to inspire you to adopt this kind of diet for weight loss and the other health benefits that it entails.

This book features chapters dedicated to some of the most frequently-asked questions about fasting. You will also learn about several myths regarding it, as it's only by uncovering the truth that you become capable of making an informed decision.

Chapter 1 – What You Need to Know about Fasting

Did you know that humans can survive without food for more than three weeks? Fasting means that you won't eat for a period of time. Intermittent fasting means that you will practice this at irregular intervals. There are different kinds of intermittent fasting, also referred to as IF, which vary with the period of intervals or the covered hours of your eating window.

IF is an umbrella term used to refer to the different kinds of diet programs that have a cycle that comes in between a fasting period to an eating period. Fasting is not a new concept. Fasting is considered a religious practice by many, including those that follow Christianity, Islam, and Buddhism. Fasting is an ancient practice that offers many health benefits aside from weight loss.

Many people who are trying to lose weight have one question regarding IF though – when will you eat? The idea here is similar to falling from the top of an eight-storey building. Falling straight to the ground will definitely kill you, but if you fall with someone catching you at each floor, the result is going to be different. The total distance of the fall may be the same, but the impact is not.

The concept of falling from a building is similar to the foods that you eat – they will boost the levels of your insulin to varying degrees. In order to sustain your health and prevent insulin resistance, you have to keep the levels of your insulin low. When you fast, it heals your body and helps you lose weight at the same time.

Do not mistake fasting for starvation. These are two different concepts because with the latter, you are involuntarily deprived of food. The matter is out of your hands – it's something that you can't control, unlike with fasting.

You may not be aware, but you actually do fasting every day. This was how the term, breakfast, came about. It is the meal that is intended to break the fast that you voluntarily subject yourself to while you sleep.

Where did the idea of fasting originate?

It was said that Hippocrates, the father of modern medicine, prescribed fasting to his patients. The reason was summarized to what he has written, "To eat when you are sick, is to feed your illness." There were other known people in ancient history that supported the practice of fasting, such as Plato and Aristotle, and the Greek historian and writer, Plutarch, who believed that it is better to fast than take medicines. The founder of toxicology, Philip Paracelsus, also supported fasting and wrote that the process is the greatest remedy. The idea was supported by one of the founding fathers of America, Benjamin Franklin, who wrote that fasting is one of the best medicines, along with resting.

Many ancient Greeks observed nature and patterned their medical treatments based on their findings. They believed that people have a thing called "the physician within". They don't eat when they are sick. People (and even animals) act instinctively when they are not feeling well. These ancient Greeks also concluded that fasting helps in boosting a person's cognitive skills.

Have you ever binged on food? How did it make you feel afterwards? After having a feast and getting yourself quite full, do you feel good and energetic, or is it the other way around? More people will likely feel tired and sleepy after eating too much. This comes as a result of how your system reacted to getting too much food. When this happens, more blood is pushed to your digestive system and only a little of the blood goes up to your brain. This is actually dangerous and can even lead to food coma.

Fasting is also associated with religious practices, although it may be called by different names (such as purification and cleansing). It was a shared belief of Buddha, Muhammed, and Jesus Christ that the practice has healing powers.

Fast Facts about the Process
The 2014 review that was done by Valter Longo and Mark Mattson, and was published in the journal, Cell Metabolism, revealed that fasting helped in improving the conditions of the animal models used in the tests. These conditions include sensitivity to insulin, high blood pressure, and inflammation.

According to studies, any kind of diet that involves fasting has to be done along with a plant-based or calorie-restricted diet, in order to gain more health benefits from the process. One of these studies was done by the head of the National Institute on Aging's neuroscience laboratory, Mark Mattson in 2003. He concluded that a calorie-restricted diet resulted to lower levels of glucose and insulin in the blood (do note though, that he conducted the study on mice).

Scientists have been studying the link between reduced calorie intake and fasting as far back as the 1930s. Through time, a lot of evidences emerged, pointing out that reducing calorie consumption by up to 40 percent can extend a person's lifespan. Eating less, especially as you age, can reduce your risk of developing common health problems.

Before you undergo any kind of IF diet though, make sure that you are monitored by a physician, especially if you intend to fast for more than a day. There may be changes in your circadian rhythm and gastrointestinal system that need to be checked to ensure your safety and health.

The IF diet dictates when you should eat and not what you ought to eat. It is more of an eating pattern and it is still up to you what kinds of food you will have during the period.

Chapter 2 – What Happens to Your Body When You Fast?

When you perform fasting, the hormones in your body naturally adjust to the process. As a result, you will experience the following:

1. A boost in growth hormone secretion

This hormone in your system is responsible in increasing the availability of fats that the body can use as fuel. It also aids in preserving the density of your bones, as well as your muscle mass. A common problem that people experience as they age is the decreased secretion of this hormone. This problem is addressed through fasting, which acts as a potent stimulus to hormone production. The secretion of growth hormone can actually double after five days of fasting.

2. More energy

How does that happen? How can you have more energy when you are not eating? Your adrenaline increases as your body experiences an increase in metabolic rate. The added energy is needed to find food, and to get more food after the fast is over. During the process, the body transitions to burning fat instead of sugar for energy. In effect, you are feeding your system with your own fat or the food that it was able to store when you were not fasting or during the hours that you are allowed to eat.

3. Sustained health

You need not worry about malnutrition even if you have chosen to follow a fasting method that will take longer than the other kinds. The fat stores in your body are enough to sustain your health. It is possible for the levels of your potassium to go down a bit, but it will still remain on safe and healthy levels even if you continuously fast for two months. The levels of other nutrients in your body, such as calcium, magnesium, and phosphorous will remain stable.

Besides, you can take a multivitamin supplement to meet your recommended allowance of micronutrients daily.

4. Decreased levels of insulin

Since all foods cause a rise in your insulin levels, it only goes to say that avoiding food will cause the opposite effect. Your body will then burn fat, which will maintain the normal levels of the glucose in your blood. This effect can already be felt after a day or two of fasting, but if you want to see a dramatic reduction in your insulin levels, then you would have to do longer-duration fasts.

The Benefits of Intermittent Fasting

Given the growing popularity of intermittent fasting, a lot of people are discovering its benefits. As it continues to be known in many parts of the world, it is also beginning to attract some doubters. The fact is, this kind of diet will only work if you will do it along with the right diet and proper exercise. The diet can make you feel better about yourself, so you will live better and longer.

Here are the other benefits of the IF diet:

- Lower levels of LDL cholesterol and triglycerides
- Lower risks of oxidative stress, problems in your DNA and lipid
- Decreased chances to develop cancer
- Lower blood pressure
- Boosts your system's fat-burning capacity
- Release of growth hormone at the latter part of the fast
- Improved cellular repair and turnover
- Better blood sugar control
- Better function of your cardiovascular system
- Improved appetite control
- Protection against neurotoxins

IF affects your hormones and cells. Once you begin with the diet, the fat stored in your body becomes more accessible. Your cells will automatically undergo repair processes and you will:

1. Experience changes in your gene expression, which will give you protection against a lot of diseases and therefore, will make you live longer.

2. Have improved insulin sensitivity, which will lead to lower insulin levels. This is why fat stores become easier to access and address.

3. Undergo repair processes by removing the old and damaged proteins that have been stored in your cells.

4. Enjoy increased muscle gain and accelerated fat loss (mainly due to the greater availability of growth hormones).

IF is beneficial to your overall health and it also improves your brain function. As you continue with IF, your mental capacity will get a boost as the hormone BDNF in your brain increases, as proven by by the 2011 study about dietary restriction, done by Mattson, Duan, Guo and Lee. This hormone aids in the growth of new nerve cells. It helps the brain to function better. It also gives you protection against Alzheimer's disease. This is the reason why many people are raving how the diet can lengthen one's lifespan.

These are only some of the changes that you will experience as you fast. You have to be prepared for more, especially if this is your first time to do it. You might find it hard at first and you might not have the energy to continue doing the normal things that you do. Instead of giving up without giving it a try, this should challenge you to move forward and expect greater changes. You have to think that these changes will later lead to weight loss and improved health.

IF Helps You Lose Weight
Among its many benefits, more people are getting interested in the diet because of its capability to help you lose weight. It leads to the automatic reduction of your calorie intake since you will be having fewer meals. Weight loss is facilitated as the diet changes your hormonal levels. Your system will release the hormone that is called norepinephrine, which is responsible in burning your fats. Even when you resort to fasting for a short period of time, your metabolic rate will increase up to 14 percent. The claim was fortified in a 2015

study by Verpeut, Gotthardt, Yang, Yeomans, Bello, Roepke, and Yasrebi.

You can only imagine what more benefits can you gain when you stick with the diet for a longer duration. You only have to get used to it. Try its different variations until you find the one that will work for you. The kind of diet that you ought to follow will depend on your lifestyle. If you are often involved in physical activities that are tiring and challenging, you cannot suppress your system from food for a long time. It needs to feed on something in order to function well.

Weight loss happens as you take in fewer calories since you are eating less. As a result, your system will burn more calories than how much you are taking in. Studies have shown that IF can actually lead to about 8 percent of weight loss for 3 up to 24 weeks, which is already a big deal when compared to other kinds of diet programs.

Among the body fats that you will lose, around 7 percent will come from your waist circumference. It means that you will lose a significant amount of fat around the belly and the organs that surround it, which will result to decreased chances of developing related diseases. You will also have fewer muscle loss, unlike the other kinds of diet that require restriction in your calorie intake.

It is important to take note that you might likely binge on foods with high-caloric content during the periods that you are allowed to eat. This comes as a result of suppression, especially if you used to indulge a lot in these foods. If you will allow this to happen, you will only regain the weight that you have already lost and your body might find it harder to lose more weight.

You are what you eat and what you do. Fasting will not work on its own. You have to be dedicated and be certain that you remain disciplined all throughout. This kind of attitude is important not only with IF, but with any kind of diet techniques. The success and failure of your diet depend a lot on your attitude. For now, you have to learn as much as you can about the diet. This way, you will know how to counter the side effects and know what to do when cravings strike.

Chapter 3 – The Common Myths about Fasting

No matter what you do, many people will try to dissuade you and tell you about the myths that they have accepted as infallible truths. Here are the most common myths that certain cynics of the diet believe as truths:

1. Eating frequently, even in small portions, can reduce hunger.

There are people who believe that having frequent snacks will take your mind away from food and your cravings. While this may be true for certain individuals, there are studies that proved otherwise. Actually, the results of different studies are mixed. There are some which hinted that it can cause reduced hunger, but there are also studies which proved that it can boost one's hunger levels. It was concluded that it really varies among individuals. You cannot accept the myth as truth without trying first what will and won't work for you.

There are those whose hunger levels are best reduced by having three meals that are rich in protein than six smaller meals of the same kind.

2. You will get fat when you continually skip breakfast.

It has always been said that breakfast is the most important meal of the day. This is why many people perceive that there is something special about it that you would miss out on when you are fasting. The myth is that skipping this meal often could lead to excessive hunger and boost your cravings, which will eventually lead to weight gain.

A study done in 2014 by the researchers at the University of Alabama debunked the myth. After 16 weeks of observing more than 200 obese and overweight adults who were grouped into two (those who eat breakfast and those who don't), it was found that this factor isn't that important to weight loss. Similar to the first myth, whether or not skipping breakfast will help you lose weight also depends on individual characteristics.

3. The brain will not function well without a good supply of glucose.

There are people who aren't keen on the idea of cutting out carbs from their diet. This is based on the fact that the brain uses glucose as fuel. You have to understand that the body is a work of genius. It will make its own glucose if it lacks the supply. This is done through the process of gluconeogenesis. This is rarely needed because the body has stored glycogen in your liver. This is used to give your brain its needed fuel for several hours.

When you fast for a long period and you take in only a little amount of carbs throughout the duration, your system will burn fat and turn them into ketone that will provide the needed fuel for your brain.

Take note though that there are certain individuals who feel hypoglycemic when they fast. If you are part of this group, you have to eat small portions of meals several times throughout the day. It is also important that you seek your doctor's advice before changing anything with your diet.

4. Snacking is good for your health.

Eating often or snacking can actually increase your risk for certain diseases. This is especially true when you snack on foods rich in calories. This can lead to a boost in your liver fat, which will raise your risk of fatty liver problems. There are also studies, which proved that eating often will make you more at risk of colorectal cancer than those who stick to regular meals or the ones who fast from time to time. These studies include the recent one published in the Nature journal. It was headed by Omer Yilmaz, an assistant professor at the Massachusetts Institute of Technology.

The body can function well for hours or days without food, but it is not natural for the body to be constantly fed. There are evidences, which point that short-term fasting causes autophagy. This is a cellular repair process, where the cells utilize the longstanding protein in your system for energy. This leads to a lot of health benefits that include the protection against Alzheimer's disease, cancer, and aging. Fasting, in general, has good effects on your metabolic health. This is better and healthier than snacking often.

5. Your body will be in starvation mode when you fast.

Adaptive thermogenesis or starvation mode happens when the body reduces the calories it burns. While this may be true, the situation happens no matter what kind of weight loss technique you employ. There are even evidences, which point out that your metabolic rate will increase when you do short-term fasts. The topic was extensively discussed by Martin Berkhan, an expert about IF, on his blog. By engaging in IF, there will be a boost of norepinephrine in your blood. This will trigger fat breakdown and accelerate the metabolic process.

6. The body has a limit in the amount of protein that it can take per meal.

You might have heard from some people that the body can only digest up to 30 grams of protein in every meal. They recommend that you eat after every couple of hours in order to gain muscle. Well, that claim is not supported by any research. The fact is, that the body can take much more than 30 grams of protein, which you can take according to the eating frequency you prefer.

7. You will lose muscle when you follow intermittent fasting.

There is no evidence that proves this claim. Your body will burn some of your muscles as fuel no matter what kind of diet program you follow. It was even concluded in some studies that intermittent fasting may help in maintaining muscle mass while on a diet.

8. Intermittent fasting causes overeating.

Many critics of the diet argue that you won't lose weight when you fast because when you are allowed to eat, there is a tendency that you will eat a lot due to hunger and the feeling of suppression. While it is true that many dieters tend to eat a little more than usual after fasting, they only do so in order to compensate for the calories that they have lost. For as long as you have your mind set to what you intend to achieve in this kind of diet, you will always remember not to overeat during the hours that you are allowed to break the fast.

Intermittent fasting is effective in helping you lose fat. A 2014 study entitled, *Intermittent Fasting vs Daily Calorie Restriction for Type 2 Diabetes Prevention* (written by Kristin Hoddy, Adrienne Barnosky, Krista Varady, and Terry G. Unterman), proved that fasting for 3 up to 24 weeks could result to an 8% reduction in body weight and a huge decrease in the fat around the tummy. This is equivalent to 0.55 pounds of weight loss in a week. You can lose a lot more (about 1.65 pounds every week) by engaging in alternate-day fasting.

9. Intermittent fasting is bad for your health.

There are a lot of studies which can prove that the opposite is true. You can gain a lot of health benefits for as long as you fast properly and you do it along with the right diet and exercise. It improves your metabolic health, reduces your susceptibility to heart disease, and enhances your body's sensitivity to insulin.

Your brain will also benefit from the process as it boosts the levels of your BDNF, or the brain-derived neurotrophic factor. As a result, you will have fewer chances of having brain problems and depression. This kind of fasting is good for your health in general. It is also acknowledged as one of the most powerful tools for weight loss.

You are already on the right track by trying to learn more about intermittent fasting. Do not allow these myths to hinder your progress or make you lose sight of the more important benefits of the program.

What are the main perks of engaging in IF?

Intermittent fasting is beneficial in general. It is recommended for people who are intent about losing weight, gaining back their confidence, and getting back in shape and in good health. Many people prefer this kind of diet because it is easy to follow – the rules are lenient, and there are no expensive supplements involved.

Simple and effective – these are the two words that best describe IF. Many people who have gotten over the myths and have tried IF concluded that it carries the following pros:

1. Can you imagine how much money you're going to save because of the meals that you have skipped or the dine-outs that you have refused to be part of? You don't need any fancy meal during your eating windows either. The beauty of it all is that you will benefit from the process despite its simplicity.

2. The diet scheme is flexible. It is up to you to choose the days and time that you are most comfortable with.

3. You don't have to overdo the process if you can't commit to fasting longer than 24 hours. Listen to your body and follow what it says.

4. How does it feel to continually plan what you will eat for a day or for a week? There are times when you will be in the mood to do it, but there will also be times when it would feel dragging. When you are fasting, you'd have plenty of time to plan how you intend to break each fast. The meals are simple and there is no need to fuss over them. It is even better if you can teach yourself to eat the same food each time.

What are the downsides of this kind of diet?
There are some people who find it hard not to eat for long hours. This is a common problem that happens in the beginning. Consider this as a challenge that you have to get over with. Look forward to the health benefits that you will gain from the process once you have gotten accustomed to the scheme of things.

It is normal to have less energy after trying it for the first time. The idea here is that you must not get discouraged, but do your best to get the hang of things as fast as you can.

Chapter 4 – The Different Methods of Fasting

It is never too late to lose weight. There is no right or wrong time to feel good about yourself. You can do it any time you want. Always remember that whatever kind of diet program you have chosen to follow, the beginning is always the hardest. You simply have to go for it and try out your chosen technique. This will give you ample of time to find out which diet plan won't work and which one suits you best.

IF is as simple as it sounds – you will take in few to no calories for the period of time that you have chosen to fast. The idea here is to choose the type that will suit your lifestyle. Do not force yourself to commit to anything that you cannot religiously follow. This way, there will be higher chances that you will stick to the diet until you have maximized its benefits. The fasting method ought to make your life easier. You have to choose the method that will not make you feel like you are missing out on something.

Intermittent fasting can be categorized into two types – short-term and long-term. Here's a look at the short-term fasting methods:

1. The 12-hour intermittent fasting
This is considered normal and only a little adjustment is needed to follow this kind of fasting every day. It requires three meals each day that you will eat during the hours that are included in your eating window. For example, you have chosen the eating window to fall in between 6AM to 6PM, this means that you will fast and avoid eating anything from 6PM to 6AM. The fast will be broken with a light breakfast.

This kind of fasting is good enough to lose a little weight and avoid obesity. Make sure that you avoid consuming excessive amounts of sugar and unprocessed food.

2. The 16-hour intermittent fasting

This is also done every day. The fasting period will happen for 16 hours, which will leave you with an 8-hour eating window. Many of those who follow the diet choose to skip breakfast each day. The usual time that is allotted for the eating window is from 11AM to 7PM and fasting will begin from 7PM to 11AM.

The method was further developed and later on, popularized by Martin Berkhan, which named it after his website. This is the reason why it is sometimes referred to as the LeanGains method. This is best suited to those who regularly go to the gym and are intent in building muscle and losing fat.

For women, it is recommended to fast for a period of 14 hours per day. Men, on the other hand, should aim for 16 hours. You can eat within the remaining 8 to 10 hours. Make sure that you don't get any calories during the fasting period, but you are allowed to have diet soda, black coffee, sugar-free gum, and calorie-free sweeteners. Most followers of this diet fast through the night, and break it at around six hours upon waking up. You have to make sure that you can stick to the schedule before you commit to it because disrupting the process can affect hormone function.

It is also up to you when to begin the fasting. You should start it depending on the time that you usually work out. What do you eat after the fast? If you will hit the gym after the fast, you have to take in more carbs than fat. On the days that you will take a break from exercising, it is recommended to take in more fat. What will remain the same is your protein consumption. It has to be fairly high each day.

No matter what IF method you have chosen to follow, make sure that you get your calories from whole and unprocessed food. You can also eat a health bar or a protein shake as a meal replacement once in a while, especially if you don't have the time to prepare your own meals.

Many people find it easy to stick to this diet plan since in most days, meal frequency is not relevant. Those who follow it break their feeding time into the three major meals, squeezing them into the periods in which they're allowed to eat.

The downside of the program is that it is stricter with what you can eat because you have to prepare meals that will match the kinds of exercises you often do. It could also be difficult to plan your meals depending on your workout schedule.

3. The Warrior Diet

This is recommended for serious and devoted individuals who can commit and follow the rules. As a warrior or a follower of this diet, you will be required to fast for 20 hours each day and break it by eating a large meal at night. What you eat will contribute to the success of the program so you ought to be careful with your choices. Your body needs essential nutrients, but make sure that you consume foods that are suited for night eating. The 20-hour fast is not that strict. You can actually eat a small serving of fruit or vegetable. In short, the fasting period requires that you under-eat, which is the opposite of what you will do when it is already time to eat. The 4-hour eating period each day can be spent in overeating.

The idea here is that your system will maximize the fight or flight response of your Sympathetic Nervous System during the hours that you are fasting. This will boost your energy, will help you become more alert, and will lead to greater fat burn. The time that you are allowed to eat will maximize the ability of your Parasympathetic Nervous System to help your body recharge and recuperate. This period gives you time to relax and it also aids in digestion.

When you eat at night, your body produces hormones that it utilizes to burn fat during the day. It is important to have a fill of specific food groups during the period that you are allowed to eat. If you are still hungry after you have had a meal that's nutritionally varied (or complete), you can add a little carb into your diet.

Many people like this method because having snacks during the fasting phase is allowed. It makes it easier to adjust to the diet, especially if you're the kind who finds it hard to keep hunger at bay.

The downside of the method is that the types of food that you are allowed to eat after the fast is limited. This will make it hard for you to adjust if you love eating or you always go out with your friends. You always have to remind yourself about what to eat and in what order. The strict guidelines are hard to follow for certain individuals. This is even harder to follow for people who aren't used to eating big meals at night.

If you think that the short-term methods are not helping you attain your weight loss goal, you can try any of the following longer methods of intermittent fasting:

1. Eat Stop Eat
This type is recommended to healthy eaters who want to learn how to practice self-control. This fasting method allows you to eat your favorite foods, but you cannot take as much as you used to.

To get this done, you need to fast for 24 hours once or twice in a week. You cannot eat anything during the fasting period, but it is okay to drink calorie-free fluids. After the 24 hours that you have fasted, you can go back to how you usually eat as if nothing happened. This all boils down to timing. How do you want to end the fast? You can finish it in time for a normal meal and prepare something big and appetizing. You can also end the fast with a light snack in the middle of the afternoon. It all depends on your schedule and preference.

How will it work? The diet will only restrict how often you eat, but it won't limit what you want to eat after the fasting period. The time required for the fasting period is enough to reduce your overall calorie intake. To make the diet work, you have to do regular workout sessions, particularly resistance training. This will trim you down and improve your body composition as well.

The program is actually flexible. You cannot avoid food completely for 24 hours, especially if you are still not used to it. You will give your body the chance to get used to it before you fully commit to this kind of IF. On your first day, it is recommended to listen to your body – find out how far you can go without eating. Go as long as you can without food, but once the craving strikes, go back to eating and stop once your hunger has been satisfied. You can gradually add hours to your fasting period. To make it easier to decide when to begin the fast, choose a date and time when you are not that busy, you won't do too many physical activities, and there are no social gatherings that you are required to attend.

The best thing about this method of IF is that you are not forbidden to eat specific kinds of food. This is easy to follow since you are not required to count calories or restrict what you eat after you have fasted. If you are intent on losing weight, you have to set portions in what you eat. You have to practice eating in moderation. You can also impose the changes gradually in order to give your body enough time to adjust.

What's the downside of the diet? There are certain people who find it hard to go without calories for 24 hours straight. Not a lot of people can easily carry on doing the things that they ought to do without food. Not having anything to eat, especially for an extended period of time, make certain people suffer from side effects that include dizziness, headache, and irritability. It is also tempting to binge on food after fasting for long hours. You have to practice self-control and help yourself to easily adjust to the process. Eventually, you will get used to it and will have lesser episodes of side effects.

2. Alternate Day Fasting

This is suited for those with strict discipline about their diet and those who are intent to achieve their ideal weight. The rules are easy for this IF method – eat a little for a day and eat like how you normally would the following day. For women, the rule is to stay within 400 calories during the fasting period. For men, the limit is 500 calories.

To make it easier for you to stick to the diet, especially during the fasting period, it is recommended to have meal replacement shakes that you can consume throughout the day rather than splitting your food into small meals. Taking these shakes is only recommended during the first two weeks of the diet program. On the third week, you have to teach your system how to adapt to eating real food during the hours that you need to fast. The following day after the fasting period, you can go back to how you normally eat. After that, you will fast again and then eat normally the following day – continue until it becomes a routine. If you frequent the gym, make sure that you choose a schedule that matches the days when you are allowed to eat normally.

This is ideal for people who are serious about losing weight. By cutting your calorie intake, it is possible to lose up to two and a half pounds every week.

The downside of this program is that you might be tempted to binge on food when you are allowed to eat. If you want to maximize the benefits of the program, you have to impose self-restriction with what you eat and how much, especially during the days that you can eat whatever you want.

3. Fat Loss Forever

This is highly preferred by those who frequent the gym but always look forward to their cheat days. This combines the best parts of many IF methods, plus, you'll get a cheat day every week, which is then followed by 36 hours of fasting. The next day will be split into the different protocols of the various IF methods.

It is normal to get shocked with the 36-hour fasting rule. Many fear that they cannot keep up with it. To make it easier for you, it is recommended to time this rule during the days when you're usually extremely busy. By focusing on how to be productive and how to finish the tasks that you have already started, you can get your mind off from hunger and your cravings.

This method requires that you sign up for a program and follow a 7-day plan. The plan will be based on your age, weight, and physical activities. A timetable will be designed depending on your workload and how much weight you intend to lose.

The downside of the program is that the cheat days can actually backfire on you. It is important to eat in moderation even when it is your cheat day. If you will not impose self-restriction, it might be hard for you to go back to eating less or eating nothing at all.

4. The 24-hour intermittent fasting

This has many similarities to the Warrior method of fasting. It also allows a 4-hour eating window. Technically, fasting will last for 20 hours. You can choose the fasting time depending on which suits you the best. Some people do it from breakfast to breakfast, while others prefer fasting from dinner to dinner. It means that you will have one meal each day.

This is beneficial and healthier, especially to people who are taking medications. They can take their meds after they have eaten during the allotted period. This method of fasting is relatively easy to adopt. You can, for example, take your one meal in time for dinner, which you can have with your family. No one will notice that you have skipped breakfast and lunch. This will also work if you are an extremely busy person. You can begin the day with a cup of coffee, get busy with work, and then recharge when you get home in time for dinner.

Allow Your Body to Adjust

No matter what method you have chosen to follow, it will not be easy to get adjusted to the process. It is important to start slow and allow your body to get used to the changes before you fully commit to that plan.

Fasting is not suited for everyone. You have to tell your doctor about it if you are suffering from any medical condition or if you are undergoing special diet programs. You must also plan ahead before you commit to the process. Make sure that you are ready in all aspects, especially with the food that you ought to consume after the fasting phase.

Chapter 5 – Essential Tips to Make the Diet Work

Here are some tips that will make it easier for you to begin with any IF method and stick with it:

1. Keep yourself hydrated by drinking plenty of water. This will make you feel full even during your fasting hours. It will make it easier for you to stick to your diet program. Begin your day by drinking water first thing upon waking up. You may have noticed that you typically feel hungry in the morning. The reason for this is the lack of water intake while you were sleeping for 8 hours or so. For weight loss purposes, the ideal amount of water that you ought to consume upon waking up is at least half liter. For men, it's important to drink up to 4 liters of water daily. For women, 2 liters is enough.

2. When planning for your fasting schedule, make sure that most of the time that you will spend fasting will be done at night while you sleep. This will make it easier for you to keep your mind away from food, avoid temptations, and lessen your cravings.

3. It is better to start fasting when you are busy. This will keep your mind away from eating because you will be more focused on finishing your tasks and in keeping yourself busy with the things that you ought to finish. Many people are more compelled to give their best at work when they have not eaten. This is something that you have to learn as you go on with your diet.

Make a list of what you need to accomplish for each day. Finish all your routines upon waking up and get started on your tasks. This way, you can get many things done even before you are reminded of hunger.

4. Never feel like you are depriving yourself of food simply because you are fasting. You have to think of it as a break period from eating. Do not spend the fasting period thinking about what to eat when it's time to break the fast. Fill your mind with thoughts other than food. Consider this your break time not only from eating, but also in thinking about food.

5. Make sure that you don't forget to exercise. Follow exercise programs that will suit your lifestyle and the method of IF that you are following. Here's something to keep in mind though – there are certain exercises, such as cardio, which can trigger hunger. If you feel the same way, go ahead and look for other exercises that you can do to keep your body fit and to help in making you forget about your hunger.

6. Take branched-chain amino acids or BCAAs. There are evidences which can prove that taking them while you are on a diet can speed up the fat loss. The term refers to three essential amino acids – valine, leucine and isoleucine, which all come with a special branched structure. They comprise a third of your skeletal muscle. It is ideal to consume BCAA when you are under a low-calorie diet. This will speed up the loss of your visceral fat.

It is vital to take BCAAs when you are constantly training because they can help reduce muscle breakdown. The ideal consumption is around 12 grams each day. The result is maximized fat loss, leaner muscles, and greater ease in maintaining your ideal weight and shape.

7. Keep stock cubes handy. If you feel like you can't control your hunger anymore, you can always drink a stock cube soup. A quarter of the soup contains around 3 calories. You can cut it in half if you want. Many dieters take it before going to bed, so that they will find it easier to sleep because their mind won't end up focusing on hunger.

8. Avoid overeating by going for the same foods as much as you can. This will kill the excitement of looking forward to what you can have during the hours of your eating window.

9. It is up to you whether or not you will tell other people that you are fasting. If it is going to help and you are certain that you will get the needed support, then go ahead and share with them what you're trying to do. If you think that people will only question your decisions and mock you for what you are doing, then it is best to keep it a secret. You can choose the right people to share the information with. You might need them to boost your spirits whenever you feel low or you're on the verge of giving up.

10. You can drink coffee or tea whenever you feel like it during the day. Caffeine is known as a natural appetite suppressant. Make sure that you don't drink too much, or else, you might feel anxious. Well, aside from that, be sure not to drink it several hours before bedtime.

11. Never give up too soon. It is true that you have to find the right method of IF that will work for you. This can only be done through trial and error. The ideal trial period is at least three weeks. This will give you enough time to adjust and monitor if your body is going through any change. If nothing is happening or you are not really getting used to the scheme of things, then it is best to move on and try another IF method. Just keep on doing it until you have found the best method that will give you the most health benefits.

Chapter 6 – Frequently Asked Questions about Intermittent Fasting

To make it easier for you to understand and remember the important points about the process, here are the frequently asked question about it, with the corresponding answers:

1. Can everybody do intermittent fasting?
Definitely not. Similar to other kinds of diet programs, IF is not suitable for everybody. The following are not suited to undergo any IF method:

- People who are under 18 years of age
- Pregnant women and breastfeeding mothers
- Those who have recently undergone surgery
- Those who are suffering from any eating disorder
- People who are malnourished or underweight
- Those who have or are recuperating from fever
- People suffering from or have a history of serious mental health concerns
- Diabetics, especially the ones taking prescription medications

It is also not recommended for children and teens. Their bodies will undergo a lot of natural changes, so it is best that they wait until they become adults before trying IF or any other kind of diet programs. Healthy adults can undergo IF, but old people who are frail and often get sick must stay away from the process and similar techniques.

2. Can someone who doesn't have any weight problem follow intermittent fasting?
IF has many benefits aside from weight loss. The only way to determine if this is going to be beneficial to your health is to choose a method that suits you best and try it firsthand. Even though your weight is normal, your cells will still benefit

from the duration that you will allot to fasting because it boosts the maintenance and repair processes.

Aside from addressing health concerns, fasting has been advocated by many religious groups and is being followed as part of rituals and devotion. Even for those not into religion, fasting could be an excellent means of developing self-control.

3. How do you begin doing IF?
Adjusting may be the hardest part for a lot of individuals who are trying it out for the first time. You have to find ways to make it easier to begin, commit, and learn how to make it part of your lifestyle. Make sure that you choose a starting day when there are less temptation to eat. You can start the diet at the time when you are extremely busy that you'd barely think about food. You have to plan ahead and know beforehand what you will eat during the hours that you are allowed to.

4. Is it more effective to fast for consecutive or non-consecutive days?
Actually, it doesn't matter, for as long as you are comfortable doing the fast on the days that you have chosen to do it. There are some dieters, for example, who fast for two consecutive days, while others do it at the beginning and the middle of the week.

5. How long does a fast day last?
A day that you will spend fasting should actually last for 36 hours. For example, you had your last full meal on Sunday at 7PM. You will then have your fast day on Monday, which will last until 7AM on Tuesday. This is an ideal scenario since you had your last meal at dinnertime and your next meal after the fast will be in the morning. This is the reason why it is important to plan ahead when it comes to the time you'll begin and end each fast day.

6. What can be eaten during the hours that it is allowed to eat, and how often should one eat?

The number of times that you can eat per day depends on the method of fasting that you have chosen to follow. It can be one big meal at lunch, several small meals spread throughout the day, two major meals each day, and so on. You have to read how each method is done so that you can wisely choose the type that you can stick to and be comfortable with. There is no best method when it comes to this kind of diet. It varies among individuals, depending on activity level and kind of lifestyle.

Make sure that you take in sufficient nutrients, such as protein and fiber, which you can get from various food sources (including meat, veggies, and fish). There are also foods that you need to avoid during your fast days, specifically the kinds that are loaded with refined carbs and sugar. If you are intent on losing weight, then you must have prepared to drop the delicacies that you used to enjoy, such as ice cream, sweet pastries, rice, potatoes, and pasta.

You can still have some snacks, but this is not the right time to be picky. You can eat something raw to feed your hunger, such as slices of carrots, apple with skin, celery sticks, or a handful of almonds. The list may not sound as appetizing as the foods that you ought to avoid, but you will eventually get used to it. You simply have to think about the benefits of the process all the time, so that you will find it easier to commit.

For the drinks, you have to consume a lot of water in order to stay hydrated even while fasting. You can drink anything that has little or no calories, such as coffee or tea. If you want to drink any alcoholic beverage, it is better that you postpone it until your fast day is over. You must not consume too much alcohol because it's actually loaded with calories, meaning it can cause a spike in your insulin levels.

7. Are there easy ways to count calories when you fast?

To make it easier for you to plan meals with the right amount of calories, it is recommended to follow recipes with caloric values listed. You can also use free calorie counters that can be found on many websites. You will eventually get the hang of things, and you'll be able to effortlessly determine the amount of calories based on the ingredients and the quantity that you are allowed to consume.

8. Can you fast if you are not feeling well?

It depends on the cause of your sickness, but it is actually best to skip fasting when you are unwell. You need all the nutrients that you can get when you are sick in order to help yourself get better at a faster rate. You might get worse if you are not going to eat. Fasting will also cause stress. This is your body's natural response in order to prompt the repair process. While it helps during the fast days, it will do the opposite if you're sick.

9. Is it allowed to exercise when you are fasting?

Yes, but you must not overdo it and you have to listen to your body when it is time to stop. As revealed in several studies, those who exercise while fasting burn more fat. Other studies suggest that men who work out before having their breakfast was able to burn more fat than those who only exercised after the fast day. Aside from burning fat, exercising can give you a good distraction when your mind is starting to crave for food.

10. What if the method that you have chosen isn't helping you lose weight?

This is where the flexibility of the process comes in. Even when you have already started with a method, you can adjust it or choose to follow a different method if it is not helping you in attaining your goal. For one, you can add another fast day and make it, for example, 4:3. If you have already reached a plateau with the said method, you can try doing the Alternate Day Fasting or ADF.

It is more ideal that you think more about losing fat than obsessing about your weight. Instead of constantly checking how much you weigh, it is better if you will monitor the changes in your measurements, especially around the gut area, as you continue to fast.

When you are not fasting, you have to be always on a lookout with regards to the calorie content of the food and drinks you consume. Make sure that you stay away from anything that contains too many calories and sugar. It is also recommended to keep on moving a lot. It is ideal to do around 10,000 steps each day. You can use a pedometer to make it easier for you to monitor your steps. The exercise is something that you can adopt even after you have stopped fasting or have chosen to try another diet technique.

11. How often should one's weight be monitored and what is the best way to get your body's measurement?

You can get your weight at the end of each week to learn about your progress. Again, it is more important to monitor fat loss, especially around the waist area, than to obsess about your weight. To effectively measure your waist, stand with your feet apart. Breathe like you normally would and begin measuring directly against the skin, but make sure that the tape measure is not compressing your skin even a bit. The measurement must start in the middle point of the lowest rib to the top of the hip bone, almost touching your belly button.

12. Does this kind of diet come with side effects?

Similar to other diet techniques, the first side effect of this program is hunger. This is normal in the beginning while you are still giving your body time to adjust to the changes. This might be more difficult at night, especially when you are not used to sleeping on an empty stomach.

In this case, you can have a late night snack to satiate the craving. It is not likely that you'd suffer from constipation and headaches, but if you experience them as side effects, this means that there is something wrong with what you are doing.

You have to drink more water during the day in order to prevent these. There are also studies which point out that a person is likely experience the side effects that he's expecting to experience even before starting the program. In this case, it is best that you only have positive expectations when you decide to commit to the program.

Fat is energy dense. This is the reason why it takes a long time to burn, especially as you age. There will really come a time when you would need the help of diet programs and learning how to use readily-available ingredients, such as coconut oil, to speed up the process. It is important to remember that you cannot overcompensate for the nutrients of which you have deprived yourself during your fast days.

It's normal to feel shaky after fasting for several hours. There are certain people who feel like they would faint after a couple of days without food. You can counter the feeling because it's all in the mind, unless you are diabetic. For healthy individuals, it is only natural for the body to maintain proper blood sugar levels and it will keep on doing so after fasting for several days.

13. How hungry can you get?
There will be times when you will be reminded of hunger, but the moments will pass. You can help yourself get through the phase by drinking a calorie-free drink, going for a walk, or by doing anything that could provide the needed distraction.

The belief that you will be in starvation mode when you fast is only a myth. The body naturally increases your metabolic rate when your calorie intake is reduced.

14. Does fasting affect gout?
It is not likely to happen with intermittent fasting. IF can help in reducing your inflammation, which can get worse if you suffer from dehydration. Make sure that you drink lots of

fluids throughout the day while you are fasting. To lessen your risk of gout in general, consume less foods that are rich in purine, such as sardines, cauliflower, alcohol, oatmeal, liver, and lentils.

15. Is it safe to fast after undergoing an operation?
It is best not to force your body to fast a few weeks after a minor operation and around two months after undergoing a major operation. It is better if you will keep a high protein diet while recuperating in order to boost the healing process.

16. How do you monitor the changes when undergoing this kind of fasting?
Make sure that you monitor your weight and measure the changes in your waist, hips, and chest. In order to ensure that your health is okay, it is also recommended to keep track of your resting pulse rate. You can use certain devices at home in order to monitor your blood pressure, fasting glucose, and cholesterol. If you can't do it on your own, ask your doctor about it or go to a licensed clinic and get the tests done.

17. How can it be easy to maintain the weight that was lost after reaching the target?
It is best to fast a day each week after you have reached your target. Keep a calorie-restricted diet in order to keep and maintain what you have already started.

Again and again, you will hear people telling you how important it is to make fasting a way of life. Through time, you will discover how to tweak the diet in order to make it more suitable to the kind of lifestyle that you are leading. There will also come a time when you will learn how to control your cravings and know the kinds of foods that are beneficial to your overall health. You have to make the diet work for you by making it flexible. You have the freedom when to begin and end each fast. It should never inhibit with your daily routine.

Chapter 7 – Foods for Weight Loss

How do you break the fast? What are the ingredients that you need to stock up on? Here are some of the best ingredients for weight loss:

Coconut oil
Coconut oil is one ingredient that must be part of any kind of low-carb diet. This oil will help you in achieving two of the most important goals of IF – losing weight and boosting energy. What's so special about this oil and how can you use it?

- Coconut oil enhances your system's ability to digest food, speeding up the process of burning body fat. As a result, it will be easier for your body to absorb the nutrients from the food that you eat.

- It gives you more energy. This is due to its important component, which is the medium-chain triglyceride (MCT) lauric acid.

- Daily intake of coconut oil can suppress your hunger and food cravings. If you find it hard to consume the oil on its own, you can mix this with your drinks or add it to your food.

- Taking it daily can make your digestive tract healthier and more capable of absorbing fat-soluble vitamins.

- The oil helps in balancing your hormones. This will result to better digestion and improved mood, metabolism, and sex drive. The oil makes it easier for your system to burn stored fats, specifically in the problem areas, such as the tummy, waist, and thighs.

- It regulates your blood sugar levels. The oil acts on the food that you take, so your body uses a little of its digestive enzymes. Your pancreas is not overworked, and that is why it is able to produce insulin without any hassle. The oil, being a saturated fat, gets mixed with insulin upon digestion. In effect, your body gets a sufficient supply of glucose or blood sugar.

Coconut oil is now being tagged as the most weight-loss-friendly fat in the world because of its composition and health benefits. Despite this, you must bear in mind that this is still oil and it has a high calorie content. Make sure that you do not go beyond the recommended daily limit, which is three tablespoons.

You can try the following ways of including this oil into your diet in order to get your needed energy boost:

- Use the oil in preparing and cooking healthy dishes, such as salad, curry, and stir-fried or sautéed vegetables.

- Take it like how you would take a vitamin pill. Limit your daily intake to two to three tablespoons each day, especially when you are already old. Remember that the oil has energy boosting effects, so do not take this before you sleep. This will make you toss and turn all night.

- Drink coconut milk because it still contains the oil that you need. You can also try eating coconut meat.

- You can eat raw coconut, but make sure that it is mature, has a brown color, and a hard shell. This is the type of coconut where the healthy oil is obtained from.

Cutting Your Carb Intake

This is the essence of your diet. Fasting will not work if you will not cut your carb intake. Doing so will lead to a significant reduction of your hunger. Make this part of your lifestyle along with fasting, and you will automatically lose weight without the need to count calories. This is also beneficial to your health and it isn't complicated at all.

Here's a list of low-carb foods that you can mix and match or prepare in a variety of ways:

1. Eggs. This is considered among the most nutritious foods. You can use it in many dishes and it can be prepared by itself in a lot of ways. The carb content of an egg is almost zero, yet it is loaded with nutrients and healthy compounds that are good for the eye and brain.

2. Fish and seafood. They are rich in omega-3 fatty acids, vitamin B12, and iodine. Most of them have a little or no carbs at all. Here are a few good examples:

- Salmon. It contains zero carbs, but is loaded with vitamin D3, B12, and iodine. This fatty fish has a good dose of omega-3 fatty acids that are good for the heart.
- Sardines. They also contain zero carbs and are among the most nutrient-dense foods. They contain almost all kinds of nutrients that your body needs and the best thing about them is that you can eat them whole.
- Trout. This is another kind of fatty fish that is rich in omega-3 fatty acids. It also contains zero carbs.

- Shellfish. They contain small amounts of carbs, about 5 grams for every 100 grams. They are among the most nutritious foods and are loaded with nutrients.
- Other good examples include herring, haddock, tuna, shrimp, catfish, lobster, cod, and halibut.

3. Meats. All kinds of meat contain little or zero carbs.

- Lamb. This meat is loaded with nutrients, such as vitamin B12 and iron. It also contains high levels of a healthy fatty acid called conjugated linoleic acid or CLA.
- Beef. It is tasty and nutritious. It can be served in many ways and you can get this meat in various forms, such as hamburger, ribeye steak, or ground.
- Chicken. For the kind of diet that you have, it is recommended to get the fattier cuts, such as the thighs and wings.
- Pork. This is nutritious and delicious.You can also include bacon in your food list, but make sure that you only take it in moderation. However, avoid bacon that has lots of preservatives and is cured in sugar.
- Other meats you could try include venison, turkey, bison, and veal.

4. Vegetables

This diet requires that you eat your greens, especially the cruciferous and leafy kinds. Stay away from starchy root veggies that are high in carbs, such as sweet potatoes and potatoes.

- Tomatoes. These are considered fruits or berries, but are mostly eaten as veggies. They contain healthy nutrients, such as potassium and vitamin C.

- Broccoli. This is rich in fiber, vitamins K and C, and other cancer-fighting compounds. It's tasty and can be eaten raw or cooked.
- Brussels Sprouts. They have the same levels of nutrients as broccoli and can be served in a variety of ways.
- Cauliflower. This is another versatile vegetable. It also contains high levels of folate, vitamin K, and vitamin C.
- Onions. They are tasty and give a strong flavor to your dishes. Aside from that, they're rich in anti-inflammatory compounds, fiber, and antioxidants.
- Kale. This healthy vegetable contains high amounts of carotene antioxidants, vitamin C, vitamin K, and fiber.
- Cucumber. It has a mild flavor because it mostly contains water (but it does have a little amount of vitamin K).
- Eggplant. This is also a fruit that is mostly eaten as a vegetable. It is high in fiber and can be enjoyed in many ways.
- Asparagus. This delicious vegetable has a good dose of protein, and nutrients, such as vitamin C, fiber, folate, antioxidants, and vitamin K.
- Mushrooms. They contain high amounts of vitamin B and potassium.
- Bell Peppers. These are known for their satisfying and distinct flavor, and they contain high levels of carotene antioxidants, fiber, and vitamin C.
- Green beans. These legumes are loaded with nutrients, including protein, magnesium, fiber, vitamin K, potassium, and vitamin C.
- For greater variety, you may try these other veggies – Swiss chard, spinach, cabbage, celery, and zucchini.

5. Fruits and berries

Because they contain more carbs than veggies, it is important to limit your intake of fruits to a couple of pieces each day. There is an exception to the rule though. There are fatty fruits (such as olives and avocado) and berries with low sugar content (like strawberries), which you can indulge on.

- Avocado. It is a unique fruit because it contains a good dose of healthy fats and only a little amount of carbs. This is also rich in potassium, fiber, and other healthy nutrients.
- Olives. This high-fat fruit is delicious and nutritious. It contains healthy nutrients, such as copper, iron, and vitamin E.
- Strawberries. They are among the most-nutrient dense fruits. Despite containing minimal carbs, they're rich in manganese, antioxidants, and vitamin C.
- Apricots. Aside from being delicious, they are loaded with potassium and vitamin C. Also, they're not loaded with carbohydrates.
- Grapefruit. This citrus fruit is rich in carotene antioxidants and vitamin C.
- Raspberries, oranges, lemons, mulberries, and kiwi are other excellent choices.

6. Fats and oils

There are many fats and oils that you can include in your diet, but avoid refined vegetable oils that can be unhealthy when taken in excess. These unhealthy oils include corn oil and soybean oil, and the healthy and low-carb types include the following:

- Extra virgin olive oil. It is considered the healthiest fat and is rich in anti-inflammatory elements and antioxidants. It's good for your cardiovascular health and can be served as part of many dishes, including the heart-healthy meals of a Mediterranean diet.

- Butter. It has zero carb content and contains high doses of nutrients. It is recommended to choose the grass-fed type of butter.
- Other examples of fats and oils include lard, tallow, and avocado oil.

7. Nuts and seeds

Nuts can be eaten as snacks, while seeds are typically incorporated into recipes, such as salads. They are both staples of low-carb diets because they are rich in micronutrients, fat, protein, and fiber.

- Almonds. These nuts are filling, crunchy, and tasty. They are also rich in magnesium, Vitamin E, and fiber.
- Peanuts. They are loaded with vitamin E, fiber, magnesium, and other vitamins and minerals.
- Walnuts. They are delicious and contain high levels of the omega-3 fatty acid ALA.
- Chia seeds. This is included in the list of the most popular health foods in the world. They are loaded with dietary fiber and other essential nutrients. The seeds can be added to various low-carb recipes.
- You may also enjoy coconuts, macadamia nuts, flax seeds, hazelnuts, pumpkin seeds, sunflower seeds, cashews, and pistachios.

8. Beverages. You can have any sugar-free drink. Do make sure to avoid fruit juices because they are loaded with carbs and sugar.

- Water

- Tea. Different kinds of tea offer numerous health benefits.
- Coffee. It is rich in antioxidants and helps in reducing your risk of certain diseases, such as Parkinson's, Alzheimer's and type 2 diabetes. This is best taken as black, but to add variation, you can also take it with heavy cream or full-fat milk.
- Carbonated water/Club soda. This is only water with carbon monoxide. Choose the kind without added sugars.

9. Condiments and herbs. They add flavor to your dishes and they contain low amounts of carbs, but are rich in nutrients.

- Salt
- Pepper
- Cinnamon
- Oregano
- Garlic
- Mustard

10. Dark chocolate. Who says that you can't have a treat while on a low-carb diet? Just make sure that you buy real dark choco that's at least 80 percent cocoa. It is known for numerous health benefits that include lower blood pressure, decreased susceptibility to heart ailments, and healthier brain function.

11. Dairy products

Full-fat dairy is suitable for your diet, but make sure that you avoid the kinds with added sugar.

- Heavy cream. It is high in fat, but low in carbs and protein. You can take it with your coffee or with a bowl of fruits or berries.

- Cheese. It is tasty and can be used in many recipes or eaten as it is. Don't forget that it's nutritious as well. One slice of cheese contains the same amount of nutrients as a glass of milk.
- Greek yogurt. This is also called strained yogurt, which is thicker than the regular kinds of yogurt. It is rich in protein and other nutrients, but has low carb content. It also has a distinct flavor that's not ideal for snacking, so try to add it to your dishes instead.
- Full-fat yogurt. This is as nutritious as whole milk, but has added nutrients. Of course, it contains healthy probiotics. These gut microbes allow you to maximize the nutrients you get from food, and protect you from illnesses caused by the proliferation of bad bacteria.

Conclusion

I hope this book was able to help you to learn more about intermittent fasting. The details are meant to inspire you to take advantage of its benefits and start adapting the process into your lifestyle. It's now time to prepare yourself – choose a date and plan your activities to begin fasting.

As you engage in your weight loss endeavor though, be sure to note any changes in your body. While it's important to track the pounds you shed, you shouldn't overlook anything that could be a bad sign. Again, it's recommended to do IF with the guidance of a dietitian or a physician.

Thank you again for purchasing this book!

Can I Ask for a HUGE Favour?

If you enjoyed this book, found it useful or otherwise then I'd really appreciate it if you would post a short review on Amazon. I do read all the reviews personally so that I can continually write what people are wanting and help them achieve success with their fitness goals.

Thanks for your support!

Other Books By Steve Blum

Ketosis Diet: 30 Day Plan for Optimal, Super-Effective Fat Loss with Ketogenic Diet

www.ingramcontent.com/pod-product-compliance
Lightning Source LLC
Chambersburg PA
CBHW070233290526
45789CB00004B/1600

* 9 7 8 1 5 4 0 8 4 3 2 7 2 *